A Husband'  the Menopause:

Because she said I could

By

Nigel Porter

Copyright © 2024 Nigel Porter

Book Illustrator:
Somerset Artist, Mike Jackson.
ISBN: 978-1-917129-71-8

All rights reserved, including the right to reproduce this book, or portions thereof in any form. No part of this text may be reproduced, transmitted, downloaded, decompiled, reverse engineered, or stored, in any form or introduced into any information storage and retrieval system, in any form or by any means, whether electronic or mechanical without the express written permission of the author.

ABOUT THE AUTHOR

I had the fortune of being born on the picturesque Island of Guernsey. It was soon apparent I had a love for the sea, at 16 I joined her Majesty's Forces and played a very small part during the Falklands conflict in 82.

Met my extremely beautiful and very lucky wife Helen in 87, we married the same year and have lived in Somerset, England ever since. I have a passion for both Motorcycles and Woodwork and have had two furniture builds published in a national magazine.

My shooting skills acquired in the corps led me into target rifle shooting where I competed for both County, Country, and Corps! At 60 something, now like many, I've succumbed to that broken stage, where your old bod' starts letting you down, I self-medicate with humour, the support of my good lady wife, and a decent red wine!

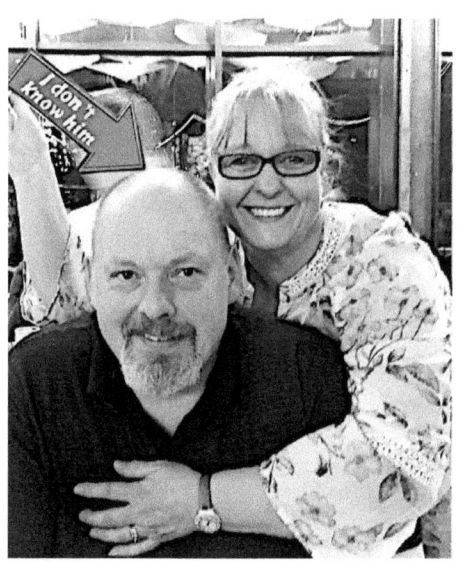

INTRO!

Being married for some 37 years, we've had our ups and downs, tragedy and turmoil, but there's always been love, laughter and humour.

This short book is directed at the very humorous side of issues raised whilst we coped with the symptoms of menopause, then interpreted with my own personal perspective of surviving most of this period (no pun) without needing to go to A&E

I hope this will put a smile on the faces of all who can relate to the content.

Foreword

I initially wrote and posted a few lines on social media with the simple intention of making my wife Helen, and both family and friends laugh. There was so much positive feedback, that I had my arm bent to turn the script into a short book, so others could enjoy!

The content is based upon the actions of my wife, whilst we (I) try to survive menopausal madness. It is my own perception of events with a comical and entertaining twist, in the hope of putting a smile on the face of all who are suffering from those magic moments initiated by our mad, crazy women!

Chapters!

1 The Beginning.

2 Countering Depression.

3 Sensory Perceptions.

4 Sleeping with the Enemy.

5 Consideration and Understanding.

6 Battle of the Bush.

7 The Crime Scene.

8 Supermarket Weep

9 Till Death Do us Part.

10 Epilogue.

1   The Beginning.

It's far too easy to go through life taking youth for granted, along with the issued 'once only' skeleton that you take on every adventure, that very human scaffolding which keeps everything in place and upright. But like any structure, it does degrade over time. So, enjoy your young bones whilst you can!

We first met in a bar where Helen worked, I was 24 the wife to be 19, we married within a year and after another had passed, we had been blessed with two bundles of joy.

Must admit seeing your little ones born is awesome; watching life coming into the world is simply amazing. Sadly, there is a downside, looking at the state of your partner shortly after giving birth is like witnessing some scrote steal your car and speed off in the distance; although you know you are going to get it back at some point, common sense tells you it's never going to be the same again.

By the time we were 20 years in, I could tell she was seizing up a bit, so I thought I would be the devoting husband she deserved, and promised I would do my best to help.

I would strategically leave underwear and socks on the floor, often in different places and sometimes partially hidden behind furniture, nothing too difficult to find as my objective wasn't to annoy.

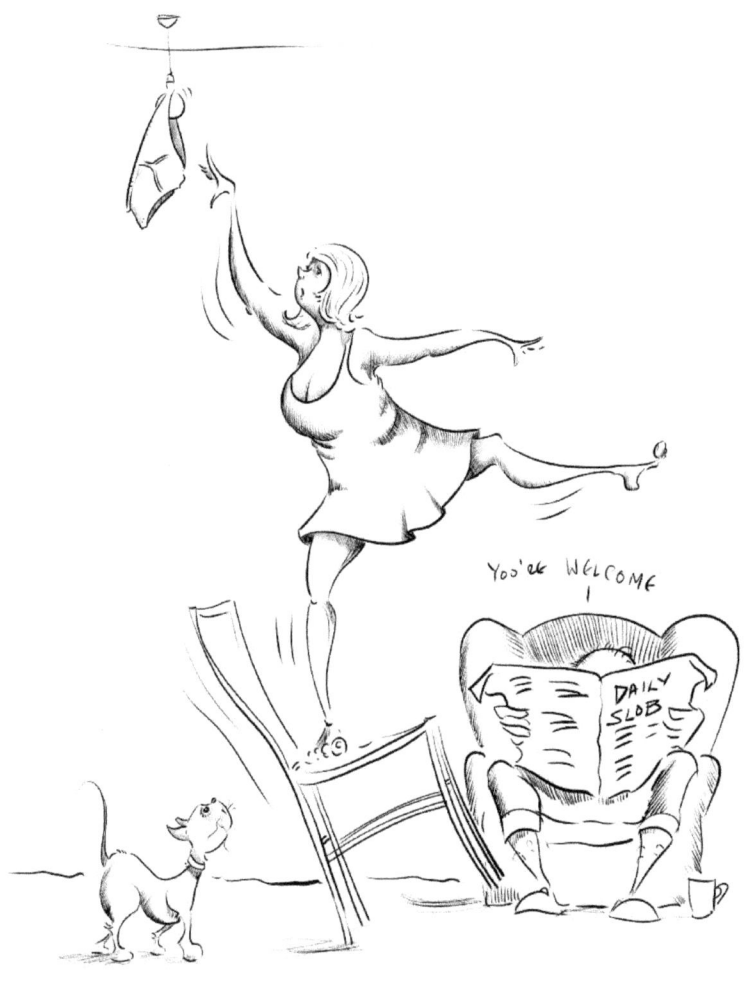

I just thought the constant bending and daily stretching would keep her spine flexible! This loving and selfless act does occasionally go unnoticed and is often mistaken by partners; but persist and think in the long term this will do them the power of good!

2 Countering Depression

There are and will be many occasions when your partner feels she simply can't cope; Witnessing these basic skills start to diminish is somewhat upsetting, as they often don't know what to do with themselves. If help isn't available at this milestone, it is very easy for the lesser of the species to fall into a numb state of mind. Beware, this can sadly lead to depression, so it's important to keep them as active as possible and make them feel needed.

I find it best to make out I've lost my keys or wallet. I then act dumb like I don't know where I've left them. Fortunately, she has a natural willingness to help; this soon turns to frustration, and it's not long before she's turned the room upside down on my behalf. Her endorphins at play during this hunt has triggered a huge sense of duty; her raised voice proves how excited she has become, and when she manages to find the lost treasure, there's a sense of overwhelming joy. This feeling of pleasure boosts self-worth and gives her great purpose in life.

Not only does this cut the head off depression, but they also know it pleases you, the husband, very similar to a dog fetching a ball. It's very important not to ignore this achievement and somewhat essential to show praise upon retrieval; either a pat on the head or a kiss on the cheek followed by a "well done you" as you ruffle her hair, goes a very long way.

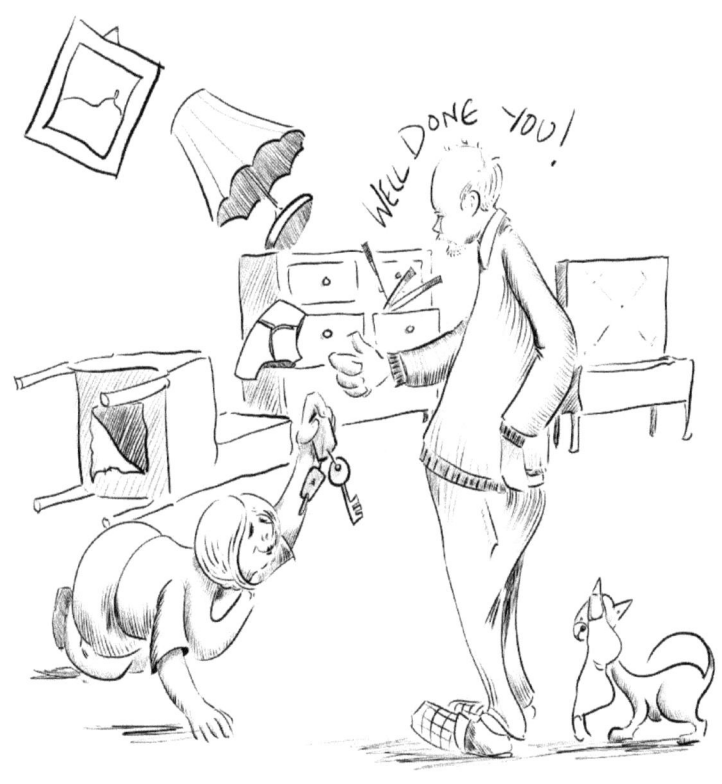

Remember, you are not only doing this to inject your loved one with self-esteem, but you are also lifting her confidence and, at the same time, giving them a sense of commitment. Do not underestimate this technique; it's essential!

But be prewarned. It is crucial to apply the above gratification with the correct amount of praise; if not, you may receive a grunt, accompanied by strange upward eye movements. If this happens, the exercise needs to be repeated with a lost phone! I know it's time-consuming, but she's worth it!

3 Sensory Perceptions

During this slightly awkward moment in her life, it's commonplace that her senses may be somewhat affected. This being the case, the husbands' efforts to please consequently go unnoticed. It's good to check these senses are in order and, at the same time, let them feel equal by making the odd mistake yourself.

Put a smile on their often-strained faces, by offering to load the dishy thingy, and throw some laundry in the washer, at the same time promising to prep a snack for later!

Put washing powder in the dishwasher so you can clean the kitchen floor at the same time as the crocks, ensuring everything gets that extra sparkle! (Genius).

Add copious amounts of tissue paper to a few trouser pockets. This will give the clean laundry an artistic twist on removal. The look of surprise on her face will be a sheer delight!

Popping an egg or two in the microwave (or a tin of beans) for a couple of minutes on high, should do the trick. You can't beat an egg sarnie or a decorated microwave!

Anticipating the somewhat pending doom, it's time to make an excuse to rapidly bolt the household. Making sure you've turned on the white workhorses, call out those magic words, "love you, see you later."

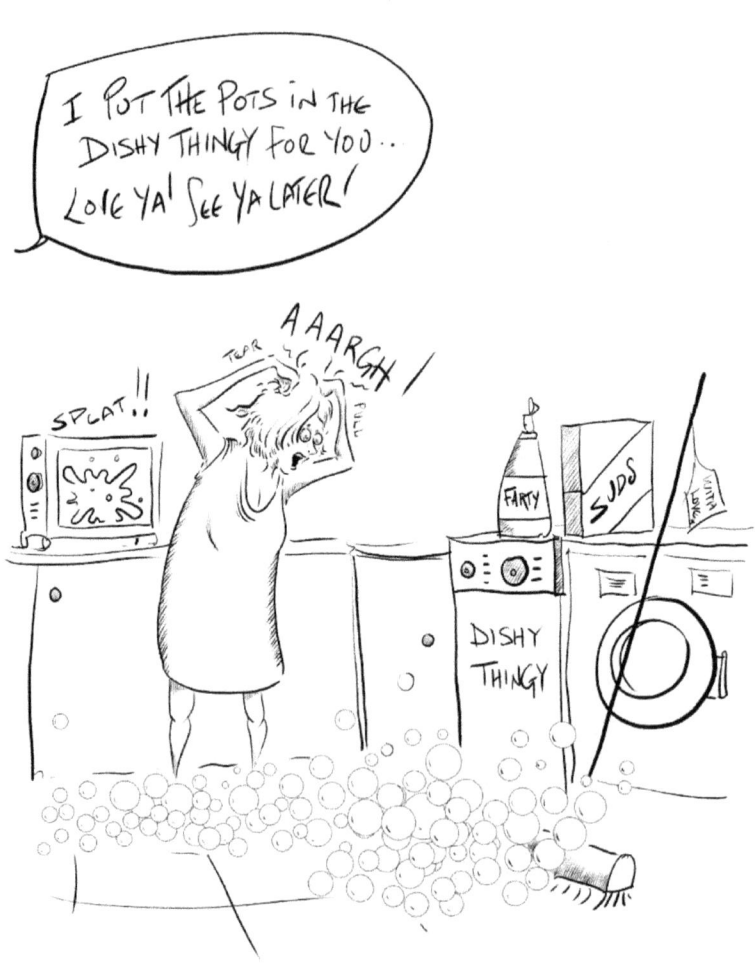

Upon returning to the loving home, it's possible there may be evidence that menopausal stress is already leaching your loved one's body. This is a good sign; however, much caution is needed here. If the change in chemistry is too rapid, objects have been known to levitate, and head in one's direction.

Whatever the consequence, keep your mind at peace in knowing it's a skill to be able to let your loved one vent. This selfless, stress-relieving technique, alongside many others, seems to come naturally to most and will add years to her life!
Bless 'em!

4   Sleeping with the Enemy

The dark hours, getting horizontal, and becoming one with the bed, this is the very best time of day. It does take a while with knackered bones to get comfy, but after necking a few meds, I'm usually pushing out the Zed's within an hour. She is doing the same but landing on the bed like a shot rhino!

It doesn't seem too long a time passes before there's an issue; it usually means me waking up with a frosty arse and ice-cold feet, as the loved one has decided to cocoon herself in an entire king-sized quilt, always happens and I can't understand why someone with the average temperature of lava does this.

Now, trying one's best to retrieve a little quilt from the sleeping dragon, I am trying at least to keep a single leg warm, and grab the cat in an attempt to delay hyperthermia.

Nerves kick in as I see an eye open, I'm laying so quiet you could hear a fly fart, it's time to keep my fingers crossed in the hope she doesn't growl, if she does, I know I've got a problem.

Currently blue with cold, but it's not an issue (survival mode has kicked in). Don't get me wrong, I can handle myself, but this is a game changer; I've broken the sleep of a menopausal monster that gets irritable and threatens instant castration if I put an arm under her pillow and try to cuddle in, there's now a need for self-preservation.

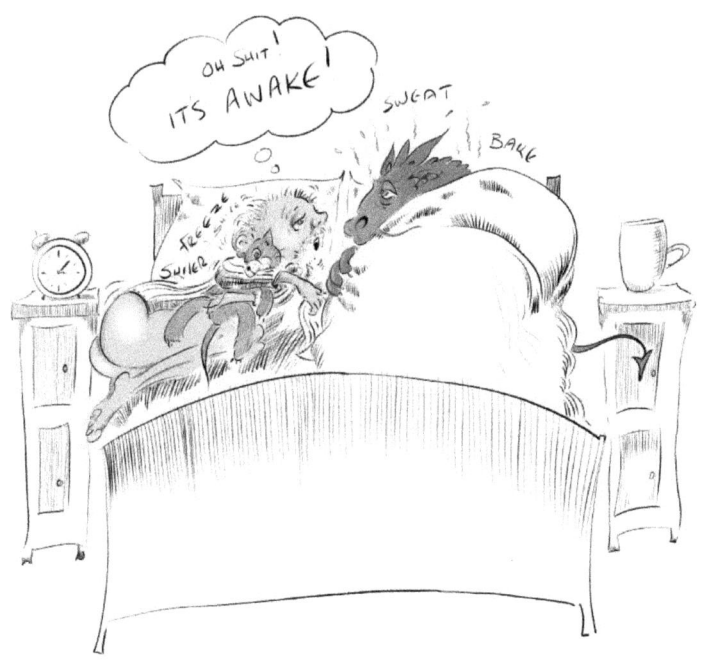

Sadly, it does seem the open eye has woken that very part of her brain, that tells her she is literally on fire.

There's something magical about lying next to an angry windmill whilst you're trying your best not to move a muscle! The skill it takes in unwrapping oneself in a nano-second and placing the entire quilt and a couple of pillows at the far end of the room is nothing but impressive. Somewhat likened to a scene out of the Matrix.

The uncovering has now released enough heat to melt a glacier, and my tits are in tatters as the cat has used me as a springboard to escape the madness!

Ten minutes of bedroom reconstruction whilst the good lady douses herself in cold water, shaves her feet, and has a dance in a cloud of talc, then we are all set for round two.

5 Consideration and Understanding

Throughout this somewhat sluggish time in a woman's life, her body isn't as efficient as it used to be, a bit like a half decent well-loved motorcycle that you enjoy riding, but sadly can no longer get spare parts for, and although you still adore it you know you're going to have to give it a hefty shove if you want to get her working. When it does spring to life, it immediately starts to cough, fart, leaks a little, then over-heats!

Remember, as with any disability you must make allowances, be considerate and take great care not to overstep! Hence, when the 06:15 alarm barks, I wait for the first-morning grunt and fart; moments later, 'Menopausal lift off' the floorboards creak (IT'S ALIVE!) Usually followed by a "Morning gorgeous' as she smacks my arse, farts again and makes a sloth-like move downstairs!

Sadly, her ageing body has played the Joker card, and since then I have noticed her struggle in the mornings, and yes everything does take a little longer, hence not wanting to cause upset or get in the way of this slow yet refined process, I unselfishly lay in bed and let her do what needs to be done, I am a gentleman after all.

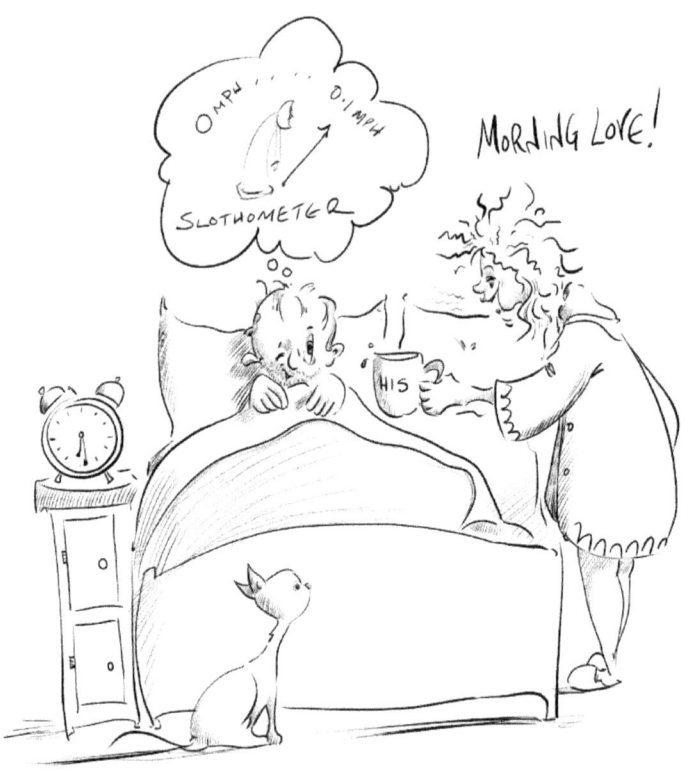

Patiently and lovingly waiting the additional 10 to 15 minutes is a struggle, but it's worth it just to see the joy in her face when she brings my morning coffee. It is indeed a beautiful moment. I am so glad I could be here for her. So, give her the time she needs. She will love you for it!

6 Battle of the Bush

It's far too easy for a relationship to become dormant, so every now and then, it's good to get out and treat the loved one, and of course have some fun.

Just need to remember, the days of surprise are long gone! Now if we go out, there's a minimum requirement of at least four days' notice, a bit like a warning order in the military.

This gives the hairy beast enough time to prep' her mindset and gather all the necessary tools needed for her to pamper herself, in the hope of creating something that is as close as possible to that gorgeous creature you managed to trap all those years ago! It will take some doing!

But that said, in the early days, it only took her a few minutes; in fact, she was simply stunning, she just had to wash her face and wipe her arse, and she was good to go!

Nowadays, some 37 years later, she's gone for ages. Maybe one of the reasons, dare I say it, is the menopausal hair growth! What used to be a neat tuft of grass is now a good half acre of brambles, and that does take time to manage. Saying that, she does have the kit to do it, whether she can complete the task on a single charge is another matter!

Then there are the legs and my knackered razor. The number of times I've gone to shave with what I thought was a new blade, only to find out it's been used as a scythe for a good 20 minutes and is now resting next to my toothbrush, wearing a wig!

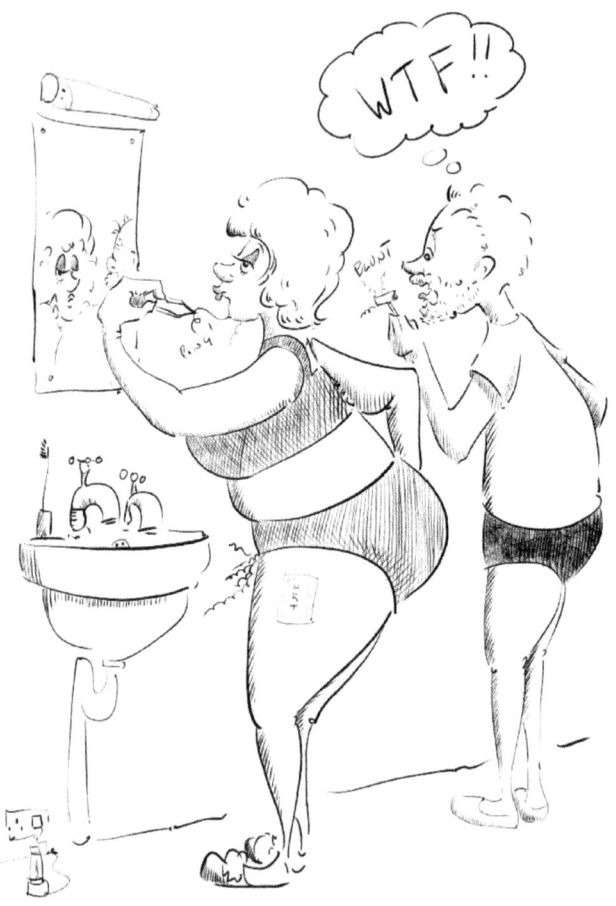

I couldn't use it anyway. The shaving mirror's never where it's supposed to be. I eventually find out it's wherever the sun was shining most the previous day. Seems that plucking anything that resembles new facial hair growth has become a daily ritual, and keeping the chin smooth is a personal battle she's not going to lose.

Finally, the colouring of the hair, and that stinky stuff that has the same smell as rotting eggs, I can't fault the commitment. If I had to smell like a fart for 25 minutes every-time I had my hair clipped, I'd look like a hippy now!

Three hours have passed, she's not dressed yet!

7   The Crime Scene!

Something is amiss in the household, it's almost like a 'who's done it' murder mystery, the bathroom door is half open, and there's what looks like the remnants of a furry beast on the shower floor. As I'm ranting, the cat has a puzzled yet somewhat bemused look on his face, he's probably wondering what all the fuss is about (he's been blamed before).

With caution, I approach the corpse with rubber gloves and loo roll, old military skills are starting to kick in, as I'm not entirely sure what this thing is, or even if it's dead or alive? It's looking like a mega rat, with what seems to be a smaller cadaver clinging onto the toilet seat! If alive, Boris the cat is getting man handled and locked in the loo, until the killing is finished.

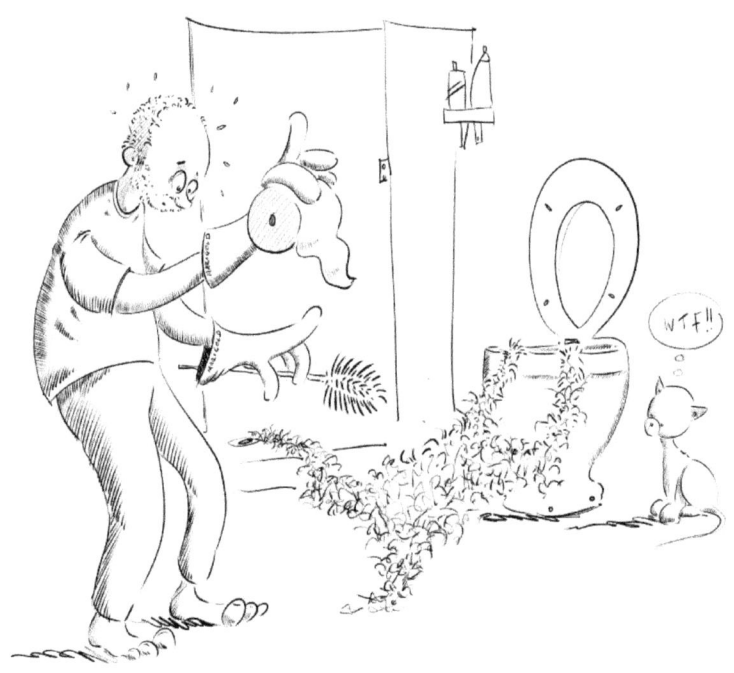

On closer inspection there's no heartbeat, the furry beast and his accomplice are in fact a good half kilo of the wife's' hair, which she's pulled out of the plugs after disemboweling both shower and sink traps. I swear that bloody cats laughing.

The changing room we have now looks like a chemist's store, she has every box of sanitary product you could mention, but something's amiss, the floor is white, and the air is misty, it looks like a scene from Narnia!

I can just see through the air and I'm now choking, I reach for a gasmask I haven't got, then realise I'm not dying or being gassed, I'm simply chewing on airborne Talcum powder! It looks like she's thrown a bottle of the stuff at the fan and done a star jump, in the hope it lands on places she can no longer reach!

Fortunately, I can follow the guilty party as there's white footprints heading towards the staircase, thinking to myself she's probably looking for the new HRT patches, as she's got to stick one on her arse every 3 days. The white footprints continue down the stairs, through the living room toward the kitchen and utility, where she's caught fighting with what looks like Casper the ghost, eventually she wins the battle, as last night's sweaty victims the sheets and pillowcases, are stuffed into the washing machine. She turns her head and growls at me, "you men are so lucky, you lot don't have to put up with this shit", I play the trump card and say a single word "COFFEE!"

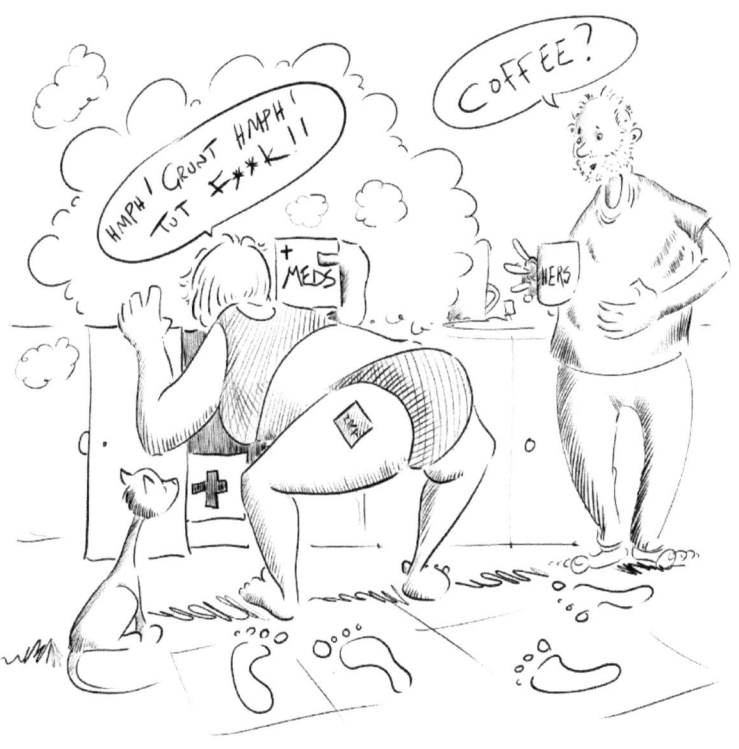

Then, with white feet and patched arse she trundles to the kitchen drawers, turning everything out as she's forgotten exactly where she has left her morning meds, she's now like a wild pig hunting truffles in a forest! A few minutes of burrowing pass, until her nasal senses sniff out her menopausal stash. Although successful, she once again starts to burn up.

It could now be the middle of winter; she doesn't care, she's opened every door and window, in the hope the house can suck in some cool air! She's in what we call danger mode, (mid hot flush) she's that hot she could toast bread.

A while later she's a tad calmer, it seems the 25mph wind blasting through the house has done its job. She's now sat with feet up, a coffee in one hand, and phone in the other. I now need to prep' my ears for 2 hours of calls to family and friends about HRT and lady problems. Happy Days!

8 Supermarket Weep

This weekly event generally starts with the 07:00 banging of cupboard doors, be it the fridge, freezer or food cupboards; she is checking our food stock like we are approaching some form of apocalypse, bending over into the depth of cupboards with her arse in the air shouting out what we need, at the same time expecting me to remember each and every item, or at least write it down. At this moment, she realizes I'm not even in earshot, I am in fact, in the loo taking care of morning business, and wondering if what has just left my body is some form of world record!

As if by magic, I appear in the kitchen with cleansed hands, and somewhat fulfilled with a sense of personal achievement. I immediately get scowled at, and have a pen and pad lobbed in my direction, followed by a scorning look that kickstarts her inventory process for a second time.

A good 15 minutes later, she's done and stands up from the lower freezer compartment, groaning and creaking like an old barn door. She then insists on checking our now comprehensive list to make sure I've not forgotten anything or indeed added anything; I then get told I haven't written this out in isle order for the supermarket (CAN'T WIN). Handing me back the pad to rewrite, she says I'm going to get dressed and drags her aching body upstairs!

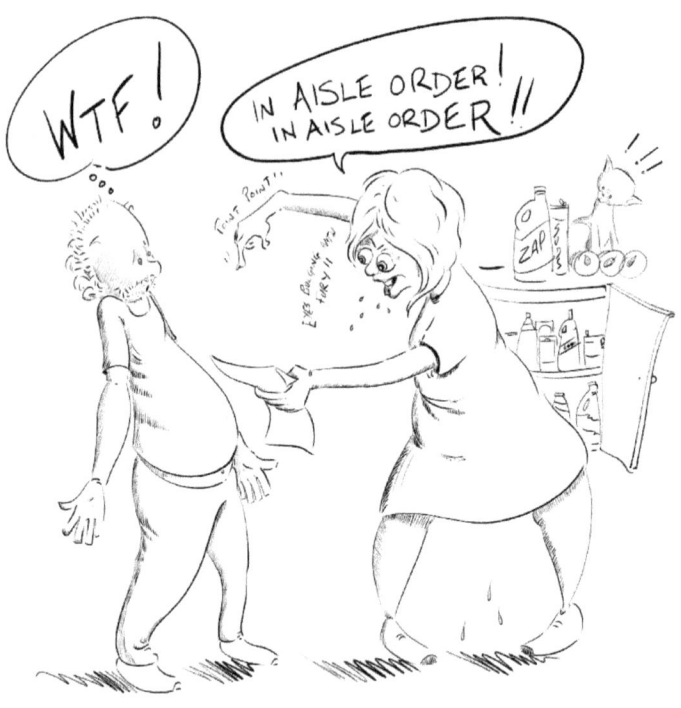

On-route to the store, I get reminded not to drive over any bumps or potholes; she's always about 30 seconds away from wetting her pants. I can't help giving her what I think is a funny light (and loving) finger dig just below the ribs. This immediately ignites a death stare. Somewhat regretting my last action, I decide to make sure the car is well out of the gutter; by doing this, I sadly and unknowingly (honest) managed to hit every cat's-eye marker in the middle of the road. I now get told if I ever want sex again, I better start driving properly. Surprisingly, the car starts behaving itself!

On arrival, it's a brief opportunity to demonstrate that cars can be reverse parked, quite simply and with ease. I find myself wanting to point out this fact verbally, but recalling the loving finger dig, and the fact that I've already chanced my luck once already, I manage to swallow my words, and stop them leaving my lips.

After a somewhat graceful yet awkward vehicular disembarkation, she must now find a trolly she can navigate. As per normal, the first three go in every direction but straight; these get put to the wayside for others to struggle with, fortunately, the fourth gets her approval, and off we go!

On entering the supermarket it's obvious we have picked the wrong day; the store is rammed, so to make life a little easier we grab a "scan and go," and head straight to the fresh foods aisle. As soon as we get there, we have a problem, we're stuck, can't move an inch, half a dozen shoppers accompanied by a couple of pensioners, all have trolleys which seem to have been abandoned, all oblivious to the carnage they're causing, and chatting away without a care in the world.

We are properly jammed, can't even backtrack. There's now a build-up behind us, with people thinking we are part of the problem. I know this will wind up my better half, and I can see she is clearly struggling. Her polite yet direct *"Excuse me"* growl goes unnoticed, and straight away, the tell-tale signs of menopausal rage are starting to show; the white knuckles you usually see on a roller coaster ride are now apparent and locked onto the trolley, her face is red, and she's now wearing that blank Mike Tyson' stare he used to show, just before the bell rings.

I do know all isn't lost, and there's still time to avoid the need of a first aider; the last warning sign will be when her ears start to wiggle. If this happens, I've got two choices: I either deny all knowledge of knowing her, and slope off without her noticing, or I rugby tackle her to the ground before she kicks off, starting a bust-up I simply cannot win. I now have butterflies in my stomach and admit to feeling a tad nervous, (I'm shitting my pants) as I just don't know how this is going to pan out.

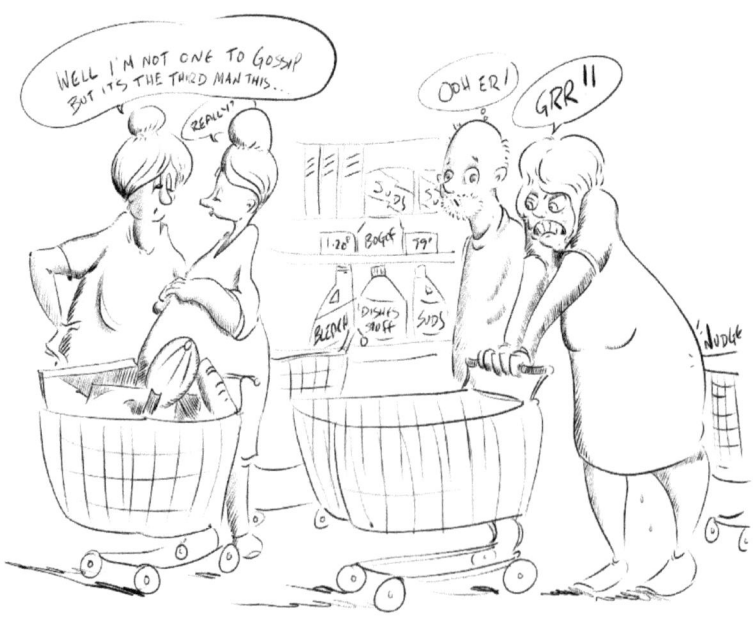

Her second growl is a tad louder; fortunately, the biggest guy hears this familiar beast-like warning, whilst also noticing both snarling teeth and drool running down her hairy chin. With haste he grabs his trolley and moves on as fast as his feet will carry him, giving me a sympathetic nod as he passes. Thankfully his disciples follow him, panic over!

Now the good lady is free from traffic, but she's already reached boiling point; we've only been here five minutes, and she desperately needs to cool down. She takes herself off to the loo, she's undoubtedly gone to have a pee and douse her face in water, also needing to take a few moments to calm herself, and get rid of the wolf-like facade.

She's had funny looks' before when she's done a balancing act on the edge of a store freezer, leaned over, and face-planted a family pack of frozen peas simply to cool her face.

Leaving me with the responsibility of the scanner and metal cart, I know I can't move, and must discipline myself to stand guard, stupidly, I've done my own thing before, I've been in this exact situation, but abandoned the trolley and took the scanner with me; This was in the foolish belief that I had some form of sanctuary within a food store. Wrong after 10 minutes, I was found and beaten with a French stick and a bag of crusty rolls (Note: crusty rolls and baguettes hurt but don't leave bruises)

A short while later, she appeared with an armful of sanitary products and said, "As I was passing the smellies aisle, I thought I would save some time and get these on my way."

I know I'm a bloke, but I'm almost a specialist in these products now, yet in the early days, I thought a maxi-pad was for a lass with a big fanny; I didn't realise it had anything to do with menstrual flow rate! I couldn't understand why women went from tampons to pads either; I'm led to believe it's got something to do with the pelvis and the floor.

I did once refer to the dreaded white tampon string, said it made her look like a walking party popper, and told her not to worry, as I wasn't going to detonate it. It was at that moment in time I realised how hard she could slap!

After everything was scanned and thrown in the cart, we carried on shopping. All was going sweet until I got handed the bread; apparently, deforming bread is a knack only a male has. It doesn't matter how carefully we handle this item. It always comes out looking like modern art, somewhat deformed and unrecognizable.

Watching me stuff the loaf in the trolley, she's again getting hot under the collar; needing to escape the shopping chaos, she takes charge of the chariot and pushes through shoppers, weaving in and out like a seasoned athlete. I've not seen her so agile in months and have realised the elderly can dodge a bullet also, it's either that or they're going to fall like skittles. It must be a sense of survival that they've become accustomed to and undoubtedly witnessed before, they are old, but they aren't going to be victims of menopausal trolley-rage today!

At last, we get to the checkout, an automated unmanned pain in the arse, that never does what it's supposed to do. Straight away, we have an issue, and there are at least four other red lights flashing before we get any help, and only one young lad trying to appease everyone, poor bastard!

Wifey guesses this is going to take a while and hands me her bank card, at the same time demanding I don't lose it (I think I'm on my fourth this year already). She's undoubtedly off for another pee. She returns just as the scanner issue is fixed; then she tries to get her vouchers off her phone, *NO WIFI*. She is now ranting that technology is really crap, informing everyone that life was so much easier before the introduction of these bloody machines! I'm biting my bottom lip, trying not to laugh, if I do, that baguette is going in places I don't want it to go!

With her bladder as near empty as it will ever get, the trip home was worryingly pleasant. I used these few quiet moments wondering who was going to do what, when we get home. I'm usually given the task of hauling the bags and boxes from the car to the kitchen, trying my best to stay out of the way, yet failing miserably. It's bizarre, we've been in the same house for over six years, and I apparently still don't know where anything goes.
It's a skill!

9   Till Death do us Part!

(Which maybe sooner than I think)

I remember our wedding day with fondness, it was a bit of a DIY job, but a great day. Like most of our generation we had traditional vows, none of this fluffy stuff you get these days. But looking back, I do feel something was missing.

Maybe ceremonies should come with a "caution card," not much, but just a little heads' up! Let's face it when you invest in all other white goods there's always an efficiency label.

Your vows make no comment the first 10 to 15 years, your Bride will be an A star appliance but, BEWARE in 15 to 20 you'll be lucky if she manages a D minus.

EFFICIENCY RATING

A+   B-   C   D-

Also, a memo' that the instruction manual will no longer work, doesn't matter what buttons you push, you won't be able to control it, or indeed turn the faulty goods off, can't even recycle the merchandise, as no one else will want it. Tuff shit buddy, you did the asking!

A further warning could also be given: Saying that it's more than likely your bride will change shape beyond all recognition, and that you, the husband will be blamed for it!

Perhaps, a little notice that shit's possibly going to go downhill somewhere in the middle, with a worst-case scenario that you may need to convert part of your garage into a menopausal panic room, this would have been a huge advantage.

Looking back, would I change anything? Of course not, although the goods are somewhat irreparable now, knees are knocking, and certain body parts are in different postcodes, I've sort of grown somewhat attached to the old growler.

I also have a sixth sense with her now, which took years to refine, I know how she both thinks and feels, and can tell when she's close by, this is possibly due to the ripples in the coffee or that "Johnny's Home" feeling you get, when the hackles on your neck come alive.

Call me soppy I know, but you can't help the way your heart beats!

Epilogue

Changing thought process totally. Wondering if Dinosaur Menopause was the reason for their extinction, small brains so they didn't have the skills in negotiation, hence couldn't retreat or surrender, so just annihilated each other. Makes perfect sense, need to rewrite history! (There's a pattern here).

A few interesting facts and highlights:

The menopause erases the female ability to point a car, and or park! She learned how to drive some 32 years ago; I've been reminding her how to drive ever since. (It's a sense of duty).

We have been happily married for over 35 years, she's had migraines for 34, (I'm still working on a cure!). Wonder if I'm the problem, (NAH!).

When she says: Do whatever you want, I don't care. (She does and she's REALLY PISSED, just hide).

She will share anything apart from Chocolate and Cake. (Especially the cake, be warned forks do hurt).

When she asks does this dress make her bum look fat. (Don't recite the chocolate and cake).

Despite all the ups and down, the constant weight changes, mood swings, tearful tantrums, copious amounts of clothing stuffed in any spare space as nothing ever fits.
SHE IS MY WORLD, AND I LOVE HER TO BITS!

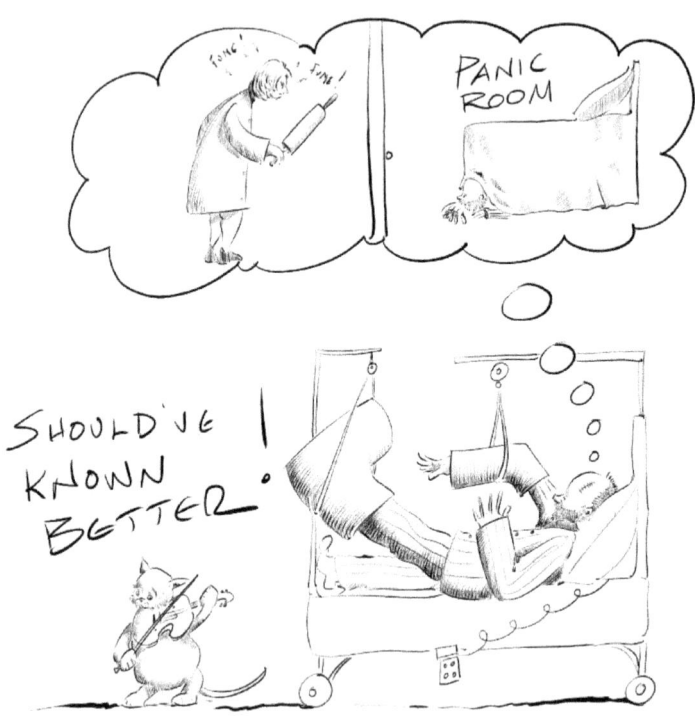

This short book was finally published and made public last Friday, I eventually made the trip to A&E the following morning!

Notes for those suffering now!

It's ok for me to have a laugh alongside Helen, but there have been some traumatic times. She had been one of the many, who's symptoms didn't show early, and when they did it led to crisis and breakdown both physically and mentally.

It wasn't until this very moment in time, that we knew she desperately needed help. So please if you are struggling and believe you are going through this most difficult of times, do get help from your GP as soon as you can.

Getting the correct medication to replace hormone levels and maybe counselling to understand why you have become a gibbering wreck is essential. Helen was off work for some time before she was fit enough to return. Fortunately, her work was extremely supportive.

A large percentage of women end up walking away from the workplace and isolate themselves, where in most cases this could be avoided, as help is out there.

Don't be a statistic, please ask for help!

Milton Keynes UK
Ingram Content Group UK Ltd.
UKHW020652290424
441924UK00015B/814